Contents

INTRODUCTION

The ketogenic diet is a very low-carb, high-fat diet that shares many similarities with the Atkins and low-carb diets.

It involves drastically reducing carbohydrate intake and replacing it with fat. This reduction in carbs puts your body into a metabolic state called ketosis.

When this happens, your body becomes incredibly efficient at burning fat for energy. It also turns fat into ketones in the liver, which can supply energy for the brain.

Ketogenic diets can cause massive reductions in

blood sugar and insulin levels. This, along with

the increased ketones, has numerous benefits.

The diet is currently being used to treat several

types of cancer and slow tumor growth.

KETOGENIC DIET FOR CANCER

The ketogenic diet is a very low-carb, high-fat

diet that shares many similarities with the Atkins

and low-carb diets.

It involves drastically reducing carbohydrate

intake and replacing it with fat. This reduction in

carbs puts your body into a metabolic state

called ketosis.

When this happens, your body becomes incredibly efficient at burning fat for energy. It also turns fat into ketones in the liver, which can supply energy for the brain.

Ketogenic diets can cause massive reductions in blood sugar and insulin levels. This, along with the increased ketones, has numerous benefits.

 The keto diet is a low-carb, high-fat diet. It lowers blood sugar and insulin levels, and shifts the body's metabolism away from carbs and towards fat and ketones.

DIFFERENT TYPES OF KETOGENIC DIETS

There are several versions of the ketogenic diet, including:

Standard ketogenic diet (SKD): This is a very low-carb, moderate-protein and high-fat diet. It typically contains 75% fat, 20% protein and only 5% carbs (1Trusted Source).

Cyclical ketogenic diet (CKD): This diet involves periods of higher-carb refeeds, such as 5 ketogenic days followed by 2 high-carb days.

Targeted ketogenic diet (TKD): This diet allows you to add carbs around workouts.

High-protein ketogenic diet: This is similar to a standard ketogenic diet, but includes more protein. The ratio is often 60% fat, 35% protein and 5% carbs.

However, only the standard and high-protein ketogenic diets have been studied extensively. Cyclical or targeted ketogenic diets are more advanced methods and primarily used by bodybuilders or athletes.

The information in this article mostly applies to the standard ketogenic diet (SKD), although many of the same principles also apply to the other versions.

There are several versions of the keto diet. The standard (SKD) version is the most researched and most recommended.

The diet is currently being used to treat several types of cancer and slow tumor growth.

OTHER HEALTH BENEFITS OF KETO

The ketogenic diet actually originated as a tool for treating neurological diseases such as epilepsy.

Studies have now shown that the diet can have benefits for a wide variety of different health conditions:

Heart disease: The ketogenic diet can improve risk factors like body fat, HDL cholesterol levels, blood pressure and blood sugar.

Alzheimer's disease: The keto diet may reduce symptoms of Alzheimer's disease and slow its progression.

Epilepsy: Research has shown that the ketogenic diet can cause massive reductions in seizures in epileptic children.

Parkinson's disease: One study found that the diet helped improve symptoms of Parkinson's disease.

Polycystic ovary syndrome: The ketogenic diet can help reduce insulin levels, which may play a key role in polycystic ovary syndrome.

Brain injuries: One animal study found that the diet can reduce concussions and aid recovery after brain injury.

Acne: Lower insulin levels and eating less sugar or processed foods may help improve acne.

However, keep in mind that research into many of these areas is far from conclusive.

A ketogenic diet may provide many health benefits, especially with metabolic, neurological or insulin-related diseases.

FOODS TO AVOID

Any food that is high in carbs should be limited.

Here is a list of foods that need to be reduced or eliminated on a ketogenic diet:

Sugary foods: Soda, fruit juice, smoothies, cake, ice cream, candy, etc.

Grains or starches: Wheat-based products, rice, pasta, cereal, etc.

Fruit: All fruit, except small portions of berries like strawberries.

Beans or legumes: Peas, kidney beans, lentils, chickpeas, etc.

Root vegetables and tubers: Potatoes, sweet potatoes, carrots, parsnips, etc.

Low-fat or diet products: These are highly processed and often high in carbs.

Some condiments or sauces: These often contain sugar and unhealthy fat.

Unhealthy fats: Limit your intake of processed vegetable oils, mayonnaise, etc.

Alcohol: Due to their carb content, many alcoholic beverages can throw you out of ketosis.

Sugar-free diet foods: These are often high in sugar alcohols, which can affect ketone levels in some cases. These foods also tend to be highly processed.

Avoid carb-based foods like grains, sugars, legumes, rice, potatoes, candy, juice and even most fruits.

FOODS TO EAT

You should base the majority of your meals around these foods:

Meat: Red meat, steak, ham, sausage, bacon, chicken and turkey.

Fatty fish: Such as salmon, trout, tuna and mackerel.

Eggs: Look for pastured or omega-3 whole eggs.

Butter and cream: Look for grass-fed when possible.

Cheese: Unprocessed cheese (cheddar, goat, cream, blue or mozzarella).

Nuts and seeds: Almonds, walnuts, flax seeds, pumpkin seeds, chia seeds, etc.

Healthy oils: Primarily extra virgin olive oil, coconut oil and avocado oil.

Avocados: Whole avocados or freshly made guacamole.

Low-carb veggies: Most green veggies, tomatoes, onions, peppers, etc.

Condiments: You can use salt, pepper and various healthy herbs and spices.

It is best to base your diet mostly on whole, single-ingredient foods. Here is a list of 44 healthy low-carb foods.

Base the majority of your diet on foods such as meat, fish, eggs, butter, nuts, healthy oils, avocados and plenty of low-carb veggies.

A SAMPLE KETO MEAL PLAN FOR 1 WEEK

To help get you started, here is a sample ketogenic diet meal plan for one week:

MONDAY

Breakfast: Bacon, eggs and tomatoes.

Lunch: Chicken salad with olive oil and feta cheese.

Dinner: Salmon with asparagus cooked in butter.

Breakfast: Egg, tomato, basil and goat cheese omelet.

Lunch: Almond milk, peanut butter, cocoa powder and stevia milkshake.

Dinner: Meatballs, cheddar cheese and vegetables.

WEDNESDAY

Breakfast: A ketogenic milkshake (try this or this).

Lunch: Shrimp salad with olive oil and avocado.

Dinner: Pork chops with Parmesan cheese,

broccoli and salad.

THURSDAY

Breakfast: Omelet with avocado, salsa, peppers,

onion and spices.

Lunch: A handful of nuts and celery sticks with

guacamole and salsa.

Dinner: Chicken stuffed with pesto and cream

cheese, along with vegetables.

Breakfast: Sugar-free yogurt with peanut butter, cocoa powder and stevia.

Lunch: Beef stir-fry cooked in coconut oil with vegetables.

Dinner: Bun-less burger with bacon, egg and cheese.

Breakfast: Ham and cheese omelet with vegetables.

Lunch: Ham and cheese slices with nuts.

Dinner: White fish, egg and spinach cooked in coconut oil.

Breakfast: Fried eggs with bacon and mushrooms.

Lunch: Burger with salsa, cheese and guacamole.

Dinner: Steak and eggs with a side salad.

Always try to rotate the vegetables and meat over the long term, as each type provides different nutrients and health benefits.

You can eat a wide variety of tasty and nutritious meals on a ketogenic diet.

HEALTHY KETO SNACKS

In case you get hungry between meals, here are some healthy, keto-approved snacks:

• Fatty meat or fish

• Cheese

• A handful of nuts or seeds

• Cheese with olives

• 1–2 hard-boiled eggs

• 90% dark chocolate

• A low-carb milkshake with almond milk, cocoa powder and nut butter

• Full-fat yogurt mixed with nut butter and cocoa powder

• Strawberries and cream

• Celery with salsa and guacamole

• Smaller portions of leftover meals

Great snacks for a keto diet include pieces of meat, cheese, olives, boiled eggs, nuts and dark chocolate.

TIPS FOR EATING OUT ON A KETOGENIC DIET

It is not very hard to make most restaurant meals keto-friendly when eating out.

Most restaurants offer some kind of meat or fish-based dish. Order this, and replace any high-carb food with extra vegetables.

Egg-based meals are also a great option, such as an omelet or eggs and bacon.

Another favorite is bun-less burgers. You could also swap the fries for vegetables instead. Add extra avocado, cheese, bacon or eggs.

At Mexican restaurants, you can enjoy any type of meat with extra cheese, guacamole, salsa and sour cream.

For dessert, ask for a mixed cheese board or berries with cream.

When eating out, select a meat-, fish- or egg-

based dish. Order extra veggies instead of carbs

or starches, and have cheese for dessert.

SIDE EFFECTS AND HOW TO MINIMIZE THEM

Although the ketogenic diet is safe for healthy

people, there may be some initial side effects

while your body adapts.

This is often referred to as the keto flu and is

usually over within a few days.

Keto flu includes poor energy and mental

function, increased hunger, sleep issues, nausea,

digestive discomfort and decreased exercise performance.

To minimize this, you can try a regular low-carb diet for the first few weeks. This may teach your body to burn more fat before you completely eliminate carbs.

A ketogenic diet can also change the water and mineral balance of your body, so adding extra salt to your meals or taking mineral supplements can help.

For minerals, try taking 3,000–4,000 mg of sodium, 1,000 mg of potassium and 300 mg of magnesium per day to minimize side effects.

At least in the beginning, it is important to eat until you're full and avoid restricting calories too much. Usually, a ketogenic diet causes weight loss without intentional calorie restriction.

 Many of the side effects of starting a ketogenic diet can be limited. Easing into the diet and taking mineral supplements can help.

SUPPLEMENTS FOR A KETOGENIC DIET

Although no supplements are required, some can be useful.

MCT oil: Added to drinks or yogurt, MCT oil provides energy and helps increase ketone levels. Take a look at several options on Amazon.

Minerals: Added salt and other minerals can be important when starting out due to shifts in water and mineral balance.

Caffeine: Caffeine can have benefits for energy, fat loss and performance.

Exogenous ketones: This supplement may help raise the body's ketone levels.

Creatine: Creatine provides numerous benefits for health and performance. This can help if you are combining a ketogenic diet with exercise.

Whey: Use half a scoop of whey protein in shakes or yogurt to increase your daily protein intake. You can find many tasty products on Amazon.

Certain supplements can be beneficial on a ketogenic diet. These include exogenous ketones, MCT oil and minerals.

FREQUENTLY ASKED QUESTIONS

Here are answers to some of the most common questions about the ketogenic diet.

1. CAN I EVER EAT CARBS AGAIN?

Yes. However, it is important to significantly reduce your carb intake initially. After the first 2–3 months, you can eat carbs on special occasions — just return to the diet immediately after.

2. WILL I LOSE MUSCLE?

There is a risk of losing some muscle on any diet.
However, the high protein intake and high
ketone levels may help minimize muscle loss,
especially if you lift weights.

3. CAN I BUILD MUSCLE ON A KETOGENIC DIET?

Yes, but it may not work as well as on a
moderate-carb diet. For more details about low-
carb or keto diets and exercise performance,
read this article.

4. DO I NEED TO REFEED OR CARB LOAD?

No. However, a few higher-calorie days may be beneficial every now and then.

5. HOW MUCH PROTEIN CAN I EAT?

Protein should be moderate, as a very high intake can spike insulin levels and lower ketones. Around 35% of total calorie intake is probably the upper limit.

6. WHAT IF I AM CONSTANTLY TIRED, WEAK OR FATIGUED?

You may not be in full ketosis or be utilizing fats and ketones efficiently. To counter this, lower your carb intake and re-visit the points above. A supplement like MCT oil or ketones may also help.

7. MY URINE SMELLS FRUITY. WHY IS THIS?

Don't be alarmed. This is simply due to the excretion of by-products created during ketosis.

8. MY BREATH SMELLS. WHAT CAN I DO?

This is a common side effect. Try drinking naturally flavored water or chewing sugar-free gum.

9. I HEARD KETOSIS WAS EXTREMELY DANGEROUS. IS THIS TRUE?

People often confuse ketosis with ketoacidosis. The former is natural, while the latter only occurs in uncontrolled diabetes.

Ketoacidosis is dangerous, but the ketosis on a ketogenic diet is perfectly normal and healthy.

10. I HAVE DIGESTION ISSUES AND DIARRHEA. WHAT CAN I DO?

This common side effect usually passes after 3–4 weeks. If it persists, try eating more high-fiber veggies. Magnesium supplements can also help with constipation.

A Ketogenic Diet Is Great, but Not for Everyone

A ketogenic diet can be great for people who are overweight, diabetic or looking to improve their metabolic health.

It may be less suitable for elite athletes or those wishing to add large amounts of muscle or weight.

And, as with any diet, it will only work if you are consistent and stick with it in the long term.

That being said, few things are as well proven in nutrition as the powerful health and weight loss benefits of a ketogenic diet.

CAULIFLOWER ALFREDO SAUCE

This version of Alfredo sauce is sure to please on pasta, chicken or even a sandwich. It will be more tasty and better for you than any Alfredo you buy in a jar. Cauliflower Alfredo Sauce is delicious. Use any cheese you like for a different flavor. Can be used as a dip for vegetables to make a tasty appetizer.

CATEGORY: APPETIZERS & DIPS

INGREDIENTS

• 1 Whole Head of Cauliflower (chopped into pieces)

- 1/2 Cup Parmesan Cheese (grated)

- 1/2 Cup Fat Free Half/Half (not fat-free for

Ketogenic Diet)

DIRECTIONS

- Fill a pot with water and place Cauliflower in

for about 10 minutes.

- Check with a fork to make sure its cooked

through.

- Put into a food processor with the cheese and

half & Half

- Process until sauce is well blended

- If you want it thinner add more Half&Half.

GREEK STYLE ROAST TURKEY

Greek Style Roast Turkey is a wonderful flavor combination of zesty lemon and delicious herbs. The oregano, thyme, and olive oil will bring out the flavor of the turkey while giving it a nice crisp skin.

CATEGORY: MAIN DISH

INGREDIENTS

- 3 Lemons Zest removed & Juiced

- 3 Lemons Sliced Thick

- 1/3 Cup Olive Oil

- 1 Tsp. Thyme

- 1 Tsp. Oregano

- 1 Tbsp. Melted Butter

- 2 Minced Garlic Cloves

- 1 Onion Quartered

- Salt & Pepper

- 3 Sprigs of Fresh Parsley

- 2 Sprigs of Fresh Thyme

- 1 Sprig Fresh Oregano

- Kitchen Twine

DIRECTIONS

1. Wash and Dry turkey. Preheat oven to 350 degrees. Salt and pepper entire turkey including inside.

2. Squeeze juice of lemons into a cup and set aside. Put lemon zest into a bowl.

3. Take the lemon slices, fresh herbs tied together with twine, and onions and stick into the cavity.

4. Mix minced garlic with olive oil. Pour half of the lemon juice , half of the olive oil and all of the zest over turkey.

5. Place turkey in oven and allow to cook covered for 1 hour. Baste with remaining lemon juice, butter, and olive oil. Increase temperature to 395 degrees.

6. For the last 2 1/2 hours cook uncovered so the skin can get nice and crispy.

7. Turkey is done after it has cooked 3 - 3/12 hours or until temperature reaches 185 in the center.

8. Please allow turkey to completely rest for 10 minutes before carving to avoid a dry turkey.

PUMPKIN FESTIVE SALAD

Pumpkin Festive Salad is a perfect for the holidays and is a nice side salad that will go perfect with chicken, turkey or pork. You can use leftover pumpkin, sweet potatoes, or squash for this recipe. Leave out the crutons to make it Paleo and Ketogenic friendly.

INGREDIENTS

- 1 Bag of Romaine Mixed Salad (ex: Fresh Express)

- 1 Cup Diced Pumpkin

- 1/2 Cup Chopped Walnuts

- 1/3 Cup Croutons (optional)

- 1/3 Cup Raisins or Craisins

- 5 Sprigs of Parsley

- 1/2 Cup Diced Onion

- 1/3 Cup Rasberry Balsamic Vinaigrette

DIRECTIONS

1. Place lettuce mix, onion, pumpkin, and raisins

in a salad bowl.

2. On top place croutons and walnuts.

3. Drizzle dressing on top and toss well.

EGGNOG LATTE WITH WHIPPED CREAM

Make your own Eggnog Latte at home with this

simple recipe. Wonderful flavor for half the price

and no waiting in line forever to get a specialty

drink. You can control the amount of sugar and

coffee.

CATEGORY: BEVERAGE

INGREDIENTS

* 1 2/3 Cups whole milk

* 2/3 Cup Eggnog

* 3 Tsp. instant espresso or coffee

* 1/2 Tsp. cinnamon for garnish

* 1/4 Tsp. ground nutmeg

* whipped cream (ex: Reddi Whip)

DIRECTIONS

* Combine in a saucepan eggnog, milk, and

espresso.

* Set to medium low and allow to come to a

rolling simmer.

* Pour into mugs and squirt whipped cream on

top of each mug.

- Sprinkle each with nutmeg and cinnamon.

GLUTEN FREE GRAVY

Who says youneed flour to make gravy? This gluten free gravy has the savory taste of traditional gravy to compliment your dinner.

CATEGORY: SAUCE & MARINADE

INGREDIENTS

- 1/2 cup turkey or chicken fat

- 3 yellow onions, diced

- 3 cloves garlic, minced

- 3 cups turkey or chicken bone broth

- 1 bay leaf

- 1/4 teaspoon nutmeg

- 1 teaspoon minced sage

- 1 tablespoon butter

- 1 teaspoon black pepper

- sea salt, to taste

DIRECTIONS

- Over medium-high heat, melt turkey or chicken

fat in wide saute pan.

- Add onions and heat for 30-35 minutes until

soft and golden.

- Add garlic and cook will fragrant.

- Add a pinch of salt and stir.

- Add 3 cups broth and and bay leaves.

• Simmer broth to reduce by 2/3. This will take
45 minutes to an hour.

• Stir occasionally.

• Turn off heat and remove bay leaves.

• Add nutmeg, sage, butter, pepper and salt.

• Use an immersion blender or blender to bring
gravy to a gravy-like consistency.

• Test the thickness of your gravy.

• For thicker gravy return to pan and cook down
with occasional stirring.

• For thinner gravy, gradually add bone broth
(about 1 Tablespoon at a time) until desired
consistency is reached.

LOW CARB BISCUITS

Eating a low carb diet doesn't mean you have to cut out a biscuit. These biscuits decrease the carbs by using almond flour instead of all-purpose flour. Because they are drop biscuits they are quick and easy to make.

CATEGORY: BREAD

INGREDIENTS

- 1 cup blanched almond flour

- 1/4 teaspoon sea salt

- 1 teaspoon baking powder

- 4 egg whites

• 2 Tablespoons butter, cut into pieces

• 1 teaspoon Swerve (optional)

• Preheat oven to 400 degrees F.

• Grease a muffin tin.

• In a large bowl, whip egg whites until very

fluffy.

• In a separate bowl, mix the almond flour,

baking powder, Swerve (if using).

• Cut in the butter and salt.

• Gently fold the dry mixture into the egg whites.

• Dollop the dough into the muffin tins.

• Bake 11-15 minutes.

MASHED CAULIFLOWER WITH GARLIC

If you're looking for a paleo friendly substitute for mashed potatoes, then Mashed Cauliflower with Garlic is the recipe for you. Naturally gluten-free and dairy-free, this cauliflower dish has a similar taste to mashed potatoes that can be enjoyed by all. If you want to make this recipe Ketogenic Diet friendly, substitute the almond milk for whole milk or cream.

CATEGORY: SIDE DISH

INGREDIENTS

- 1 large head of cauliflower, cut into florets

- 1/4 cup almond milk

- 1 Tablespoon butter

- Head of garlic

- Fresh chives, chopped

- salt and pepper to taste

- Preheat oven to 400 degrees F.

- Peel away the outer layers of the garlic bulb and and cut of the very top of the bulb to expose the individual cloves. Place in aluminum foil and drizzle with olive oil. Then close around bulb.

- Bake for 25-30 minutes. Allow garlic to cool, then squeeze out cloves.

- While garlic is baking, place 2 inches of water in a pot. Once water is boiling, steam cauliflower in steamer for 12- 14 minutes.

- Drain pot and return cauliflower.

- Add roasted garlic, almond milk, butter and salt to cauliflower. Use an immersion blender or food processor to combine ingredients until smooth.

- Top with chives and pepper.

CHEESY SMASHED CAULIFLOWER

Cheesy smashed cauliflower is a perfect low carb substitute for mashed potatoes. The cream cheese, cheddar cheese and butter make this an excellent high fat option for those on the ketogenic diet. If desired, you can top the smashed cauliflower with crumbled bacon and chives.

INGREDIENTS

- 1 cup olive oil

- 12-14 garlic cloves

- 2 large heads cauliflower, broken into florets

- 4 ounces cream cheese

- 1 1/4 cups sharp cheddar cheese, shredded

- 1/4 teaspoon sea salt

- 1/4 teaspoon black pepper

- 2 teaspoons unsalted butter

DIRECTIONS

• In a sauce pan saute the garlic cloves in 1 cup

olive oil for 20 minutes or until garlic turns

golden brown.

• Remove garlic from oil and puree in food

processor until it forms a smooth paste.

• Steam the cauliflower 12-14 minutes until just

tender.

• Place in a large bowl and mash with potato

masher or fork.

• In another large bowl combine cheeses, salt,

pepper, butter and 2 teaspoons of the garlic

puree.

• Refrigerate remaining garlic puree in the

refrigerator for us to two weeks.

• Pour cauliflower on top of cheese mixture. Stir

with spoon until well combined.

• Serve immediately.

GREEN BEAN BUNDLES

Green bean bundles are a simple side dish that

give a fancy appearance to any meal. They are

made of fresh green beans bundled together and

wrapped in a slice of bacon. They are then

roasted in the oven where the flavors combine.

INGREDIENTS

- 1 lb. fresh green beans trimmed

- 8 bacon strips

- 3 Tablespoons butter

- 1 Tablespoon chopped onion

- 1 Tablespoon coconut vinegar

- 1 Tablespoon Swerve (optional)

- 1/4 teaspoon sea salt

DIRECTIONS

- Preheat oven to 400 degrees F.

- Blanch the beans 4-6 minutes.

• Wrap 15 beans in a bacon strip and secure with toothpick.

• Place on foil covered backing sheet and bake for 10-15 minutes.

• In a small skillet, saute onion in the butter.

• Add vinegar, salt and Swerve if you are using the sweetener.

• Remove bundles and place on a platter. Then, pour vinegar mixture over the bundles.

• Serve immediately.

LOW-CARB TWICE-BAKED YAMS

These twice-baked yams only use half of each yam, adding cooked pumpkin in it's place to lower carbohydrate content. Whipped up with cream cheese adds fat to the dish making it ideal for those on the ketogenic diet. To decrease carbs even more subsitute pumpkin with mashed cauliflower. To decrease calories use half the amount of cream cheese.

You can top these two different ways:

Loaded: sour cream, butter, bacon and cheese

Holiday: Nutmeg, cinnamon and butter.

INGREDIENTS

- 8 small yams or sweet potatoes

- 2 cups pumpkin

- 1 package cream cheese

- salt and pepper, to taste

- butter

DIRECTIONS

- Preheat oven to 400 degrees F.

- Place yams on cookie sheet. Cut an X on the top of each one and bake 1 hour.

- Cool 15 minutes.

- Lower oven temperature to 350 degrees F.

• Peel back the top edges of the yams. Leaving

the skins in tact, scoop out the middle.

• Set half aside for another recipe.

• Place the rest in a bowl and mash. Add

pumpkin, cream cheese and butter. Mix until

fluffy.

• Spoon yam mixture back into the skins and

back for an additional 20 minutes or until warm.

ASIAN BEEF & VEGETABLE STIR FRY

Take your leftover beef from dinner and add a

few ingredients to create a new dish. Beef &

Vegetable Stir fry has all those Asian Flavors you

like without the loaded fat or sodium.

INGREDIENTS

- 8 oz Beef Cooked & Sliced

- 2 Cups Sliced Mushrooms

- 1 Red Onion Sliced

- 1 Red Bell Pepper Sliced

- 2 Cups Broccoli florets

- 1 Tbsp. Low Sodium Teriyaki Sauce

- 1 Tsp. Lemon juice

- 1 Tsp. Olive Oil

- Cooking Spray

DIRECTIONS

1. Heat up and spray a skillet.

2. Start by sauteing the mushrooms for 3 minutes.

3. Now add the onion, peppers, broccoli, teriyaki sauce, lemon juice, and olive oil.

4. Saute for 5 minutes.

5. Stir in Beef and saute for another 6 minutes.

6. Serve warm.

ROASTED CAULIFLOWER STEAKS

Have Roasted Cauliflower Steaks as a side dish tonight. The cauliflower is so rich in flavor from the roasting you'll almost forget it's healthy.

INGREDIENTS

- 2 Cloves Garlic Minced

- 1 Tbsp. Olive Oil

- 1 Cauliflower Head

- 1 Tbsp. Lemon Juice

- Cooking Spray

DIRECTIONS

1. Preheat oven to 375 degrees. Spray baking sheet with cooking spray.

2. Mix olive oil, garlic, and lemon juice.

3. Cut center of head of cauliflower lengthwise into 3/4-inch-thick slices.

4. Place onto baking sheet.

5. Brush each piece with lemon oil mixture.

6. Roast for 30 minutes or until cauliflower starts

to slightly golden brown.

7. Remove and enjoy.

CREAMY CAULIFLOWER BROCCOLI SOUP

Have a nice warm bowl of Creamy Cauliflower

Broccoli Soup tonight. The savory cheese mixed

with veggies and creamy broth is a perfect

combination.

INGREDIENTS

- 1 Pkg. Frozen Cauliflower

- 1 Pkg. Frozen Broccoli

- 1 Container Chicken or Vegetable Stock

- 1 Tbsp. Butter

- 2 Cups 1% Milk

- 1 Cup Low Fat Cheddar Cheese (white or yellow)

- 1/3 Cup Low Fat Cheddar Cheese Shredded (for garnish)

- 1 Tbsp. Cornstarch

- 1 Cup Cold Water

1. Start by placing broccoli, cauliflower, stock, and butter into large pot.

2. Over medium heat allow stock to come to a simmer and allow to simmer for 10 minutes.

3. Pour in the milk and add the cheese. Stir so that the cheese melts and does not clump.

4. Once cheese melts dilute cornstarch in the cold water.

5. Pour water into the pot of soup. Allow to come back up to a simmer.

6. Remove from heat. Place soup in bowl and sprinkle with some cheese.

7. You can eat soup as is or place a hand blender into your pot to puree the vegetables for a creamier texture.

SAUTEED GREEN BEANS, PEPPERS & ALMONDS

Have Green Beans Almonds & Peppers as a side dish or vegan meal tonight. The nutty flavor from the almonds combined with the sweet peppers on top of green beans will have your taste buds dance in harmony.

CATEGORY: SIDE DISH

INGREDIENTS

- 1 Bag (1 lb) Green Beans

- 2 Red Bell Pepper Cut Into Strips (any color)

- 1 Shallot Diced

- 1 Small Onion Diced

- 2 Garlic Cloves Minced

- 1 Tbsp. Olive Oil

- Juice of 1/2 Lemon

- Dash of Salt & Pepper

- Pinch of Oregano

- 1/4 Cup Almonds Chopped

- Cooking Spray

1. Warm up saute pan and spray with cooking spray.

2. Drizzle with olive oil. Now start by sauteing garlic, onions, and shallots for 1 minute.

3. Add the green beans and saute for 4 minutes.

4. Now add the red bell peppers, almonds, oregano, salt, and pepper.

5. Saute for 5 more minutes.

6. Squeeze juice of 1/2 lemon on top and place onto serving platter.

7. Divide into 6 portions and enjoy.

GRILLED VEGETABLE SKEWERS

Grilling fresh summer vegetables enhances their naturally delicious flavors. Eat them with pasta or rice to create a complete vegan meal.

CATEGORY: MAIN DISH

INGREDIENTS

- 1 Zucchini Sliced

- 1 Red Bell Pepper Cut into Chunks

- 1 Green Bell Pepper Cut into Chunks

- 1 Onion Cut into Chunks

- 1 Cup Whole White or Bella Mushrooms

- 1 1/2 Cups Cherry Tomatoes

- 4 Skewers Soaked in Water

- Dash of Salt & Pepper

- 1 Tbsp. Olive Oil

- Juice of 1 Lemon

- 1/2 Tsp. Dry Italian Herbs

DIRECTIONS

1. Warm up grill (indoor or outdoor)

2. Place vegetables onto each skewer. Any order you like will be fine.

3. Continue until all vegetables are on the skewers.

4. Brush each skewer with oil. Squeeze lemon juice over each skewer.

5. Sprinkle with salt, pepper, and herbs.

6. Place onto grill and cook on each side for 5 minutes.

FIRE ROASTED BELL PEPPERS

Fire roasted bell peppers are a perfect side dish for any summer meal, and great for topping salads. You can add this to a sandwich too. The sweet and spicy flavors from the bell peppers really come through with the grilling.

CATEGORY: SIDE DISH

INGREDIENTS

- 2-3 Bell Peppers

- Dash of Salt

- Dash of Pepper

1. Place peppers onto grill on medium high heat.

Sprinkle with a dash of salt and pepper.

2. Cook on one side for 6 minutes.

3. Flip over and cook the other side for 6

minutes.

THYME SWEET POTATOES

Thyme Sweet Potatoes are made by taking

regular sweet potatoes and roasting them in a

marinade of honey, thyme and other spices. The

hint of salt will add a punch of flavor when

combined with the honey and thyme. Enjoy this

as a side dish anytime.

INGREDIENTS

- 5 Sweet Potatoes Peeled

- 2 Tbsp. Raw Honey

- 2 Tbsp. Brown Sugar

- 3 Sprigs Fresh Thyme Stem Removed

- 1 Tbsp. Canola Oil

- Cooking Spray

- Baking Pan

DIRECTIONS

1. Preheat oven to 400 degrees and spray or line your baking sheet.

2. Slice the potatoes into 1/4 Inch Strips. (fry shape)

3. Whisk together honey, brown sugar, and oil.

4. Place potatoes into a large bowl. Sprinkle with salt and herbs.

5. Drizzle the honey mixture. Toss well and place into pan.

6. Roast in the oven for 20 minutes.